LIFE *is really* SIMPLE, BUT WE INSIST ON MAKING IT COMPLICATED

CONFUCIUS

Anny's use of case histories and examples provide insight and inspiration.

Her variety of stories beautifully illustrate that her simple technique can encompass virtually any improvement you want for yourself.

Anny's approach is unique, practical, effective, and long overdue in the weight loss market.

Tori Scruton

The Four Mental Agreements
To Losing Weight

Anny Slegten

Published by
Kimberlite Publishing House
www.kimberlitePublishingHouse.com

KIMBERLITE
PUBLISHING HOUSE

The author of this book does not dispense medical advice or
prescribe the use of any technique as a form of treatment for
physical, emotional, mental, spiritual or medical problems without
the advice of a physician, either directly or indirectly. The intent
of the author is only to offer information of a general nature to
help you in your quest for physical, mental, emotional and spiritual
wellbeing. In the event you use any of the information in this
book for yourself, which is your right, the author and the publisher
assume no responsibility for your actions.

ISBN: 978-1-7752489-0-3

Book cover and logo designed by

Marietta Miller
http://www.execugraphx.com

THE KIMBERLITE DIAMOND CONNECTION

Kimberlite is a rock type first categorized over a 100 years ago based on descriptions of the diamond bearing pipes of Kimberley, South Africa.

Kimberlites are the mechanism by which diamonds are brought to the surface.

Kimberlitic rocks are the most important primary source of diamonds and the main rock type in which significant diamond deposits have been found so far.

Anny is familiar with many rocks and minerals as her husband was raised around quarries – and later worked in several mines in Canada.

Therefore, it was natural for Anny to choose kimberlite as an analogy to the soul residing within our body – as a diamond within the kimberlite.

The Four Mental Agreements to Losing Weight

By Anny Slegten

DEDICATION

This book is dedicated to Papa, who taught me to observe without judgment.

Very observant himself and a fast thinker, Papa taught me this by example and some stern lectures.

After all these years, I am still profoundly grateful to him for having instilled in me the ability to notice what is unfolding, and then observe the results or consequence of what has unfolded.

The ability to observe without judgment developed into the most important asset of my profession.

The only way to assess anything in an objective way is to go from effect back to cause.

By being right there in the moment of decision in the past, we realise the "what for" was the best decision and the best response and the best action we could have made at the time, however outdated it is now.

How come the "what for" instead of "why"?

There is a different response between the "why" question and the "what for."

Asking "why" invites an evasive round about and emotional justification, full of excuses.

When asking or looking at the "what for," we get a concrete, straight, and logical explanation.

This is the same as in history.
Criticizing past history issues is easy.
However, in twenty to fifty years, what we think are the most brilliant actions now, justice being done, will largely be regarded as stupid or horrible, the same way we criticize the past.

There are two sides to every story.

Whatever it was, understanding of the "what for" allows us to make peace with whatever or whomever we will make peace with, including ourselves.

Anny

AN IMPORTANT MESSAGE

First Europe, then Africa; North America is the third continent I am experiencing.

This results in sometimes an unusual way of explaining things. English is the fifth language I learned to speak.

It is interesting that I lost Flemish, my mother tongue, as well as German. I have a guttural Dutch/German accent when speaking English.

Now, when calling family and friends in Europe, they know it is me since I am speaking French with an English accent.

Having lived in Congo from eighteen months old until leaving for Canada at age twenty-five, once in Canada, surrounded mostly by white people, it took me a long time to recognise people, white people looking the same, according to me. As I am writing this, I realise this is sometimes still a challenge to me. Knowing if they were serious or joking when talking to me was also very difficult to figure out.

Having an accent, I have learned to spell some words when speaking.

For example, on the telephone, when giving directions to my office, I explain: "The fifth driveway on your left-hand side, one, two, three, four, five, the fifth driveway on your left hand side," since they sometimes understand "first" instead of fifth.

Most of my self-hypnosis recordings end with a prayer when I say:
"… bless your family, bless your friends, bless your pets if you have any, and that includes your houseplants."
Although I carefully pronounce houseplants, many people think I am saying husbands!

As suggested when taking excellent courses on how to write a book, I first sent a draft of *The Four Mental Agreements to Losing Weight* to six people, asking them for an honest review, wanting to make sure my message is clearly understood.

It was not easy for Ann, Beth, Colin, Pamela, Rhonda, and Sheryl to refrain from correcting some sentences, respecting my way of expressing myself.

The funniest one was an observation from Irish born Pamela. Having written word by word something said to a friend of mine whose health was deteriorating, "You are going down." Pamela corrected me explaining the correct way is, "You are going down hill." Looking at her embarrassment, I have now an idea about what "you are going down" means.

Please understand that my choice of words is directly connected to the ease of pronunciation. "Continuously," "pleasurable," and many more words are tongue twisters for me.

Have you ever attended a presentation by an author you admired and when listening to them wonder who wrote the book, a pseudo author whose name is printed on the book or someone else?

Once having read the book and then hearing me speaking in English, I want to make sure you know I am the one who wrote the book. That is the reason the book was edited the simplest way as possible.

Interesting enough, when I am teaching hypnotism and hypnotherapy, the way I am explaining things many times brings up good natured laughter as well as a good understanding of what I am explaining.

With my accent, a typical one is a prayer, when I say, "… please protect us from negative influences, regardless of the source, …"

I must say "influences," a tongue twister for me, since I have not found another word to explain what I want to convey, although some students are wondering how come I am asking to protect us from negative influenza.

Since then, the prayer was improved to:
"God, please allow only good things to come to us, …"

Yep. This is work, not walk.
I said work: W – o – r – k.

Anny.

ACKNOWLEDGMENT

A special thank you to you, my clients. You came to see me regarding many things you wanted to improve in your life.

Trusting me, sharing your most intimate stories, you revealed to me how unique we all are, regardless of a common symptom—in this case, being overweight.

The reason, the "what for," and the mental blocks that was created made you understand how true it is that we are all one of a kind.

And once having understood it all, you allow yourself the pleasure of slimming down in a healthy way, if that was truly what you wanted.

Hugs, of course!

Anny

TABLE OF CONTENTS

FOREWORD

by Dr. Rhonda M. Gibson

"THE SECRET OF CHANGE IS TO FOCUS ALL OF YOUR ENERGY NOT ON FIGHTING THE OLD, BUT ON BUILDING THE NEW."

SOCRATES

As a psychologist for over thirty years, I have witnessed many clients—both men and women—struggle with their weight. Our culture has led men, women, teens, and children to pursue an elusive goal of thinness to the point that it has become an obsession. It has led to psychological disorders that range from anorexia, bulimia, and BED (binge eating disorder) to anxiety and depression. The statistics are staggering. The single most critical factor that leads to an eating disorder is dieting.

The latest Statistics Canada report stated that obesity has now become an epidemic leader of diseases.

Personally, I started my first diet when I was ten. The memory was so clear.

I tried on my mother's wedding dress and it would not even come close to zipping up. We were the same height. I was horrified. I scoured my house and my friend's home to look for a diet book. I was too fat. Something had to be done. I found the most acclaimed diet book of the time and decided that was that.

I will never forget the first day of my diet. My mother is an amazing cook, and I loved all of her homemade baking. That night for supper, we had homemade bread and cinnamon buns. Well, the rest of the family did, and I chose to not.

I suffered and suffered! Weight and dieting was always on my mind.

Thank goodness our home scale did not need batteries or keep track of how often it was used, as I weighted myself three times a day, (with no clothes of course, as that would have added extra pounds). I struggled with my weight for forty years.

I can attest I having tried every diet that has ever been developed, exercised like I was training for the Olympics, and bought every new diet product to find a magic "how to" to keep me thin. My beliefs about my weight effected my mood, my self-esteem, and my social life (which I did not have, as I could not go out anywhere being "fat").

Fat and dieting became words I hated. Dieting worked, or so I believed. I lost the weight and was so relieved and happy with myself, only to gain it back and more when I went off my diet.

That is exactly how I met Anny. I had just moved to the Edmonton region and with all the stress of graduate school, having an amazing six-year-old son, being a single parent, and starting a new job to open a new centre led me to gain not just some weight, but a lot of weight. I found Anny, we did several sessions, and the weight came off.

This year I had the true blessing to move from client to student. Anny asked me to read a draft of her book, *The Four Mental Agreements to Losing Weight*, and after being a student, I realized that Anny's work was not only remarkable, it was a true paradigm shift on weight loss.

I was astounded, all those years of torture, depravation, mood swings (Yes, I did it—"I am at my goal weight," to depression, "I am fat again." Good thing I was not a psychologist yet or I would have self diagnosed myself with bi-polar disorder).

Anny's ground breaking approach to slimming down is not only simple and pleasurable, it is a completely different way of thinking and losing the weight in a healthy and safe manner.

Could it really be so simple? If I would had read the book, I would have thought no. I, however, have had the great pleasure of being a student of Anny's and watching her work with people, understanding the theoretical underpinning of her method.

If your true goal is to reach a comfortable weight for yourself, this book is a must. Moreover, just as I did, a very high percentage of teenagers begin their eating disorder career in their teens (90% of women who have eating disorders are between the ages of twelve and twenty-five years old, while 51% of nine- and ten-year-old girls have a higher level of self-esteem if they are on a diet).

This book is a must-have for you and your children, whatever your age or gender, Anny Slegten has, in her self-help book, provided parents a powerful defense against both obesity and eating disorders.

In a world where instant gratification is a must and thinness is the gold standard, we have now been presented a new paradigm to give hope to millions of men, women, and children plagued with disordered eating and the physical, emotional, mental, spiritual, and financial distress that comes with the territory.

Dr. Rhonda Gibson
Recipient of the Queen's Jubilee Medal
Governor General's Caring Award
St. John Ambulance Medal
Venerable Order of St. John of Jerusalem

DISCLAIMER

As with everything related to health,
PLEASE CONSULT A PHYSICIAN prior to
embarking on any health-related issues.

The Four Mental Agreements to Losing Weight are
simple to follow.

It takes an accomplished therapist to lead the client
in a superconscious state of awareness to help the
client make closure on issues relating to the mental
blocks.
Yes, you read it right: Issues relating to the mental
blocks.

Please understand that the information contained in
this book is not offered as a substitute for, or
replacement of, any therapies regarding physical,
mental, or emotional ailments.

The Four Mental Agreements to Losing Weight could make
you look at your predicaments in a different light
and allow you the pleasure to slim down in a healthy
way. After all, to quote Albert Einstein:

*"We cannot solve our problems with the
same thinking we used when we created
them."*

FIRST, LET US GET ACQUAINTED!

So, there I was.

On a bright morning, fully clothed, looking at myself in the mirror, I decided enough was enough. I felt bloated and looked bloated. And, of all things, I was thinking of having to buy a larger size of panty hose. This was the supreme insult to myself.

I had ignored the one kilo a year I was packing on. However, ten years later and 10 kg heavier, enough was enough, and off it had to go. Looking at the weight in British pounds instead of kilograms, 22 lbs made it even more catastrophic.

Sound familiar?

I decided to visualise myself wearing the little suede leather suit I loved. I had two powerful hypnotherapy sessions and off went the excess baggage.

It was easy and pleasant as I went on full automatic, doing absolutely NOTHING, letting my mind do the work.

I slimmed down in one month; first my face, which
made me look sickly for about two months, and then
my *derrière*.
I wished it went the other way.
First my *derrière*, then my face. Honest.

Being in a trance is a natural process. We are in a
trance about 95 % of the time, allowing our mind to
be impressed with what we allow ourselves to be
impressed with, usually by not paying attention to
what we allow ourselves to be impressed upon.

We are in a trance when we feel we are between
being awake and asleep and not awake—the best
time to listen to a motivational recording,
impressing our mind with a subject of our choice.

Being led in a trance by a hypnotherapist is safe
since the client knows they are led in that special
place. Once in a hypnotic trance, the client becomes
super conscious and stays in control, that they like it
or not, wishing they are not responsible of the
outcome. That is right.

From the general perception of what it is to be in a
hypnotic trance, many people think their eyes are
closed and they zonk out in a deep state of
relaxation.

From there, based on what they see on television or movies, they think I would lightly touch their forehead with my magic wand, reciting some incantation, and once back to full awareness everything would be successfully done without them doing anything.

If that is really what people believe, how come do they not line up at my door when claiming they want to quit smoking, stop drinking, cheating, gambling, biting their nails, their fear of public speaking, exam anxiety and more?

Yes, a person is in control and can be in a deep trance and not follow suggestions.

The comfort and trust of being hypnotised is in the knowing by experiencing a hypnotic trance.

As a professional hypnologist and clinical hypnotherapist in full time practice for several decades now, my clients made me aware of what works, what does not work, and the best suggestions to give them for self-improvement while in a hypnotic trance.

This is my reason to write *The Four Mental Agreements to Losing Weight* and share with you, my dear readers, the secret of slimming down in a healthy way.

No prescribed diets!
No exercise regimens!
No hard work!
Pleasant.
Simple.
Easy.

It is easy: Allow your mind to set itself on the right track and let it do the work.

Since slimming down is the *focus*, only removing the mental blocks regarding weight and then using your brain by doing something physical to prove to the mind that you mean business is the best way to go. What is so important about removing the mental blocks?

A mental block automatically gets you back to whatever it was before, as soon as you relax and stop using willpower to accomplish what you want to achieve—in this case slimming down and staying slim.

The same goes for everything, be it health, wealth, career, relationships—EVERYTHING.

===================================

THE FIRST MENTAL AGREEMENT

THE FOCUS

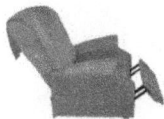

===================================

THE FIRST MENTAL AGREEMENT

THE FOCUS

One often meets his destiny on the road he takes to avoid it.

Matan Attias

There are several points to consider.
Let us first go back to the basic: The *focus*.

Yes, the first mental agreement is the *focus*.

Remember, what we *focus* on is what we get.
Therefore, what are you *focusing* on?

Without realising it, our mind creates an image of
what we think, and we then get what we think. After
all, don't we say, "I could see it coming."

So, here you are, wanting to lose weight.

Consider what you are doing since you decided to lose weight:
- Going on the scale to watch
  your weight
- Going weekly to the weigh-ins
- Watching what you eat to lose weight
- Going on a diet to lose weight
- Going to the gym to lose weight
- Exercising to lose weight

When going out:
- -Heading to the salad bar because you do not want to put more weight on.
- Choosing the lightest item on the menu to watch your weight

Just to name a few.

Even just counting your calorie intake, the 'what for,' is because of your weight!
- Watching your weight
- Wanting to lose weight

The only *focus* is weight.
Everything is about your weight.

Since your *focus* is your weight, your weight is doing well, is it not?
And you have a constant battle with your weight.

This is hard work. Who wants that? How come?

Each time you think about or mention weight, you give it life and bring it into the now.

What do you have to do to put your attention to what you want to have and then have the pleasure to have what you want to have or experience it in a pleasant way?

Thinking about "how to" is like running on a treadmill. You work hard and get nowhere.

After all, up to now how come you keep getting exactly what you do not want to have or experience?

Is it not positive to state what you do not want?

Have you noticed how children respond exactly to what you are telling them?

Say, 'Do not slam the door,' and they slam the door. How about saying, "Close the door gently."
Say, 'Do not run, and they run.
Do not cry. And they cry. Instead, how about saying, "I can tell you are not smiling."

Cigarette smokers explained that they often do not even think of smoking until they notice a no smoking sign, the one showing a lit-up cigarette with a line through it.

Also, what do we do when we lose something? We usually search for it because we want it back. Unconsciously, wanting to lose weight *focuses* on weight you want back!

It is true that eating properly and exercising responsively is good for your health. However, it does nothing for the weight except keeping it on since weight is the *focus*.

Therefore, the first thing to do is *focusing* on the pleasure of slimming down in a healthy way.

Please read this again:

Therefore, the first thing to do is *focusing* on the pleasure of slimming down in a healthy way.

The pleasure? Absolutely!

So, how come the title of the book is
The Four Mental Agreements to Losing Weight?
The *focus* is on weight!

People are so *focused* on losing weight that they would have never noticed the book had the title been "The Four Mental Agreements to Slimming Down in a Healthy Way." I am not sure that they would have found the book on line.

1 – Losing weight: "Nothing happened"

A client came to my office one day, wanting to lose weight.
Since my client was well over 300 lbs and wanting to save my recliner from destruction,
I decided to let her sit on a chair across the desk from me.

It became obvious that she was expecting me to hypnotise her to instill the regular regimen of diets and exercise. She was resisting me, ready for an argument since I was avoiding the usual belief of what to do to lose weight.

I then decided to work with her, eyes wide open. I had to bypass her belief of how to lose weight, making sure I did not perform the standard ritual first comers usually expect. You know, "Look at my fingers, listen to my voice."

About an hour later, closely observing her,
I knew I succeeded at getting her mind in the right place and decided to terminate the session.

Upon completion, my client complained,
"What? Nothing happened!"

"Well," was my response "If nothing happened, then there is no fee."

"Oh no, I am paying," was her reply. And she paid.

Back in the reception room, her friend who drove her to my office asked, "How did it go?"
"Nothing happened," replied my client.

About one month later, I started to have ladies who my client referred to me on a regular basis.

What happened?
They all told me the same thing: They could not believe how nice my client looked, slimming down, doing nothing, not understanding it since nothing had happened!

Being aware of what we *focus* on is true for everything.

How did I do this? What happened?
My students explained to me that I do not only teach hypnosis and hypnotherapy.
I also practice and teach hypnology: Hypnosis in all its form and applications.

We go into a trance, that special place all day long, even during other healing modalities, including when with a doctor or in the presence of a person we perceive as an authority figure, not realising we are in an vulnerable mental state.

Being in full time practice since 1984, I know when a person is in that special mental place. and use that door to help my clients and my friends obtain what they want, bypassing all the regular and pleasant rituals that allow them to put their guards up. This is when the mental blocks are acting up to keep the status quo, the existing state of affairs.

2 – I recently learned my own lesson

I knew my spine was in an S shape, making me lean to the left. Since I do hypnosis and know what to do, I decided to record an affirmation:

" … bring my body back to excellent physical health, my spine straight, and walking straight."

A few weeks later, as I was walking in the yard, I tripped on something. My heel went back and fell in a small hole covered with dead leaves.

I lost my balance and fell heavily on my right side. There was a loud "crack." The pain was excruciating as I yelled to the person with me, "Ken, pick me up, quick!"

Standing on my feet, in total surprise, I said, "My spine is straight!" I found out later my right hip had to be put back in place too.

Did I hear about this from my students and colleagues!

"… bring my body back to excellent physical health, my spine straight, and walking straight."

What was missing in this affirmation?
The pleasure!

The pleasure of having my body back to excellent physical health, my spine straight, and walking straight.

Yes, the pleasure. After that fall, my spine straight, hematoma healed, and my hip back into place, I had to deal with back pain due to stubborn fascia. It took massages, chiropractic adjustments, hypnotherapy, virtual hypnosis sessions, self-hypnosis recordings, and more to speed up things and enjoy my physical body again.

I keep insisting on mentioning the pleasure on the first day of the two-day "Hypnosis, an Introduction" course when I am teaching how to write and make a motivational recording or a self-hypnosis recording, all the way to the six week-long courses.

Every student who trained with me was on my back, asking how come I had not mentioned in my affirmation "the pleasure of getting my body back to excellent physical health, my spine straight, and walking straight."

They all know how often I mention and remind them of it. Here I was, me, Anny, their instructor, not having asked for the pleasure of...

When asking for something, it is important to stipulate the pleasure of whatever you are praying for or whatever you are specifying in your self talk. Other wise, you will end up having exactly what you want in the simplest way possible.

Compare how you feel when you explain, "I want to have a good job," versus, "I want to have the pleasure of having a good job."
"I want to have children," versus, "I want the pleasure of having children."

Here are a few examples, since I truly want you to understand how important is what you *focus* on.

3 – Warts

A young girl was referred to me by the family physician. She had warts all over her hands all the way to her elbows, even between her fingers. A few warts were starting to show up on her legs.

As I was interviewing her prior to starting the hypnotherapy session, she explained in great detail what had been done to get rid of the warts.
Something was rubbed on the warts to burn them off.
When eating, garlic was rubbed on the fork she was using while eating.
Even duct tape was used to rip off the warts.
This in addition to a lot of techniques I had never heard of before.

The young girl was at the age of being very careful about what she expressed, in fear of being judged.

As a result, this was a long session. We *focused* the whole time on *the pleasure of having smooth skin*, or not *having the pleasure of smooth skin*. During the hypnotherapy session, shifting the *focus* from warts to *smooth skin* was only one of the many approaches used to correct the issue.

Please understand: Mentioning having a *smooth skin* or *not having a smooth skin* creates the same image, since the *focus* is on having a *smooth skin*.

After the session, wanting the mother to keep the *focus* on *smooth skin*, I asked her mother to write down the following instructions:

At bedtime, ask the girl to drink a sip of water to have the pleasure of having a *smooth skin*.
In the morning, give her as much water as she can drink. While she is drinking the water, explain that it is to flush out everything that has to be flushed out to have the pleasure of having nice, *smooth skin*.

Within about a month, the young girl's skin was nice and smooth. No warts. No scars.

4 – Acne

In reviewing a course in hypnosis, one of my hypnotherapists had a big Ah Ha moment!

She was a single mother with two very young children. The only things she would buy for herself were products in an effort to clear her *acne*. The *focus* was the *acne*, and yes, to her amazement, her *acne* was doing very well!

Realising the same situation, another student stopped buying products for clearing her daughter's acne. Back from going shopping, the student gave her daughter a product to have the *pleasure of having a clean skin*. And the acne quickly subsided. The *focus* was *clean skin*.

5 - Accident Prone

A client called me one day in great alarm.
Although she was wrapping her car with white light for protection, she had near-miss accidents each time she was driving her car.
When asked what she was thinking when doing that ritual, her answer was, "To not have an accident."

I then suggested her to shift the *focus* from not having accident to *enjoying a safe ride*.

6 - Ah, All Those Bills to Pay

It is common to want a better paying job to pay the bills.

Low and behold, the bigger the pay, the more and higher are the bills to be paid.

The *focus* is on *bills*.

Many years ago, my husband decided we should buy a second property in British Columbia. We bought a very beautiful 65.96 hectare (163 acre) property in the Robson Valley and a new pick up truck—a must when being the owner of such a special place.

Then came moving expenses, purchasing new furniture for the home away from home, and everything needed to live in comfort. Overnight, the money in our bank account went from a lot of money to next to nothing.

So, here I was with a beautiful home away from home in British Columbia (by Canadian standards, *only* a 5 ½ hour drive from our home and my office in Sherwood Park, Alberta).

Worried at the depletion of our money, I discovered everything was multiplied by three: electricity bill, telephone bills, realty taxes, property insurance, and more. To address the situation, I decided to make a self-hypnosis recording containing the following affirmation and to listen to it when falling asleep at night:

"From now on, *all my bills are paid in full.*"

Working very hard, my income increased. About six weeks later, unexpected bills started to land on my desk.

- The wood burning forced air furnace was cracked and had to be replaced.

- The electric water heater broke down and had to be replaced.
- The new pick-up truck needed a set of studded tires.

What happened?

Having a good relationship with "Subby" (I call my subconscious mind Subby), and doing this for years, looking at myself in the mirror, I asked:

- "Subby, what am I doing to get all these *bills?*"

I could feel a silent laugh within me.

- "Subby, stop laughing. What am I doing to create all these *bills?*"

Laughing, the inner voice replied, "Look at your affirmation!"

I started to argue with Subby. After all, I am teaching this; I know what I am doing!

Subby's inner-voice repeated, "Look at your affirmation!"

By then, I cooled off and asked,
- "Subby, what is it?"

Subby, in a matter-of fact inner voice, replied, "The *focus* in on *BILLS!*"

7 - What is usually said

It is also true when you talk to someone about their weight situation. "You are not getting any *slimmer*" (The image is of *slimmer*) *focuses* on *slimming*, rather than "You are putting weight on" (The image of weight).

In a recent conversation, a friend explained "You are going down hill" was said to a person whose health is rapidly getting worse.
It would have been more helpful to have said, "You are not *getting better.*" The *focus* here is on *getting better.*

About your weight:
Do you keep searching and *focusing* on how to lose weight?

Focusing on "how to" is like running on a treadmill: You run as hard as you can and get nowhere, staying put.

How come?

The *focus* is on "how to" instead of the result: "Have the pleasure of being slim!"

When you keep thinking about your weight, "how to" and "thinking" together gives you a double whammy!

I could write more examples to ask you to start to pay attention to what you are *focusing* on. sticking to what is always on your mind.

8 - Checking my theory

Although slim enough as I am, I wanted to check this theory. One day I decided to tell myself that I had to watch myself to not get any *slimmer*. The *focus* being *SLIMMER*.

To my surprise, I started to eat a lot, my stomach yelling "enough!"
I started to slim down. Looking at how my clothes were fitting, my pants falling off when I was not wearing a belt. I guess I slimmed down about half a kilo a week.

It took me a while to figure out how to stop it.

I then remembered to establish boundaries, seeing myself wearing the little suede leather suit. My appetite went back to normal, and my clothes then started fitting me perfectly.

I love a phrase from James Allen:

"You are today where your thoughts have brought you. You will be tomorrow where your thoughts take you."

The funny part is that today is the tomorrow you were thinking and worrying about yesterday.

How true this is. We are all alchemists with the ability to materialise what we think. The stronger the emotion attached to an issue, in this case weight, the more we gain weight.

Our *focuses* are like magnets.

What we *focus* on is what we get.
It is as simple as that.

When coming for a private session, I listen carefully to my clients to detect what they keep *focusing* on.

When coming for *weight loss*, all that they are talking about is *losing weight*, and then at my request, they explain what they are doing to lose it, and the results.

Making them aware how much they *focus* on the *weight* they want to lose, the first thing is to improve how they talk about it by completely eliminating the *focus* on weight, as well as lose weight and replace it with *slim*.

Do they want to *slim down* in a pleasant and healthy way? When observing themselves in the mirror, I ask them to think, "I better start to have the pleasure of *slimming down*." The image, "Being slim or *not being slim* enough," sends the same *focus* to the mind: *slim*.

Now, let us look at you, my reader.

Please do as I do, taking notes when a client comes to my office, requesting a private session.

Complete the self-assessment about what you *focus* on, what are you obsessed about, and do this honestly.

Since writing things down by hand impresses your mind, you will have better results when writing this down by hand.

You can get a complementary copy of these questions and all the questions in this book including space to write in a downloadable PDF file at:

http://www.connectwithanny.com

Please check each question as you are writing down your answers.

Date:

_____

(1) When did you start to put weight on?

_____

_____

(2) What was going on in your life?

_____

_____

(3) How did you feel about it?

_____

_____

(4) Has anybody commented about your weight?

_____

_____

(5) What were the comments?

_____

_____

(6) What action did you take to lose weight?

_____

_____

(7) List titles of the books you read to lose weight.

_____

_____

(8) What diets did you follow?

_____

_____

(9) What club or support group did you join to lose
    weight?

_____

(10) Did you do anything else to lose weight?

_____

_____

(11) What were the results?

_____

_____

(12) What happened each time you got off the

diet(s)?

_____

_____

(13) What is on your mind when thinking of eating?

_____

(14) What is on your mind when eating?

_____

_____

(15) How often do you talk about your weight?

_____

(16) Do you have a bathroom scale? If so, how

many times are you weighing yourself, and what for?

_____

_____

What is the purpose of answering all these questions
in earnest? It is for you to be aware of what you keep
focusing on, of what is always on your mind.

Remember, what you focus on is what you get.

It is important for you to come back regularly to
these question pages to check your progress.

Please remember to write the current date each time
you record your findings.

You can get a complementary copy of these
questions and all the questions in this book
including space to write in a downloadable PDF file
at:

http://www.connectwithanny.com

Please check each question as you are writing down your answers.

Date:

_____

(1) When did you start to put weight on?

_____

_____

(2) What was going on in your life?

_____

_____

(3) How did you feel about it?

_____

_____

(4) Has anybody commented about your weight?

_____

_____

(5) What were the comments?

_____

_____

(6) What action did you take to lose weight?

_____

_____

(7) List titles of the books you read to lose weight.

_____

_____

(8) What diets did you follow?

_____

_____

(9) What club or support group did you join to lose
    weight?

_____

(10) Did you do anything else to lose weight?

_____

_____

(11) What were the results?

_____

_____

(12) What happened each time you got off the

diet(s)?

_____

_____

(13) What is on your mind when thinking of eating?

_____

(14) What is on your mind when eating?

_____

_____

(15) How often do you talk about your weight?

_____

(16) Do you have a bathroom scale? If so, how

many times are you weighing yourself, and what for?

_____

_____

What is the purpose of answering all these questions in earnest? It is for you to be aware of what you keep focusing on, of what is always on your mind.

Remember, what you focus on is what you get.

It is important for you to come back regularly to these question pages to check your progress.

Please remember to write the current date each time you record your findings.

You can get a complementary copy of these questions and all the questions in this book including space to write in a downloadable PDF file at:

http://www.connectwithanny.com

Please check each question as you are writing down your answers.

Date:

_____

(1) When did you start to put weight on?

_____

_____

(2) What was going on in your life?

_____

_____

(3) How did you feel about it?

_____

_____

(4) Has anybody commented about your weight?

_____

_____

(5) What were the comments?

_____

_____

(6) What action did you take to lose weight?

_____

_____

(7) List titles of the books you read to lose weight.

_____

_____

(8) What diets did you follow?

_____

_____

(9) What club or support group did you join to lose
    weight?

_____

(10) Did you do anything else to lose weight?

_____

_____

(11) What were the results?

_____

_____

(12) What happened each time you got off the

diet(s)?

_____

_____

(13) What is on your mind when thinking of eating?

_____

(14) What is on your mind when eating?

_____

_____

(15) How often do you talk about your weight?

_____

(16) Do you have a bathroom scale? If so, how

many times are you weighing yourself, and what for?

_____

_____

What is the purpose of answering all these questions in earnest? It is for you to be aware of what you keep focusing on, of what is always on your mind.

Remember, what you focus on is what you get.

It is important for you to come back regularly to these question pages to check your progress.

Please remember to write the current date each time you record your findings.

You can get a complementary copy of these questions and all the questions in this book including space to write in a downloadable PDF file at:

http://www.connectwithanny.com

=================================

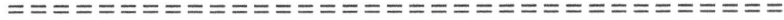

THE SECOND MENTAL AGREEMENT

DEFINING THE BOUNDARIES

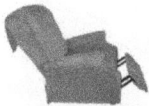

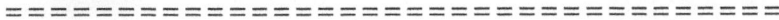

=================================

THE SECOND MENTAL AGREEMENT

DEFINING THE BOUNDARIES

I saw the angel in the marble and I carved until I set it free.

Michael Angelo

====================================

Do we need boundaries?

Yes, it is important, so you can safely reach your goal of looking and feeling great.

Looking up the word 'boundary' in the Webster's New Collegiate Dictionary, I found that a boundary is something that indicates a limit or extent.

As you want the pleasure of slimming down in a healthy way, it is important to establish limits. Otherwise, you could be unhappy about how you look, get way too skinny, and get sick as a result of it.

The same goes if you are too skinny and want to have a normal healthy looking body. In that case, you could become overweight unless you establish boundaries.

In this case, boundaries are established by the size of clothes you want to wear comfortably—looking great, feeling great.

When someone comes to see me to lose weight, having listened to check what my clients are *focussing* on and making them aware of the results, I then follow by establishing the boundaries.

This is important, so my clients can see themselves at the way they want to be in their mind's eyes. They can clearly envision the result.

What size of shirt are they wearing now?
What size of shirt would they like to wear?

What size of pants are they wearing now?
What size of pants would they like to wear?

And for ladies,

What size of dress are they wearing now?

What size of dress would they like to wear?

Having written down the size of clothes they loved to wear, looking and feeling great, I then ask them if they still have some clothes they loved to wear.

For ladies, nine times out of ten it is their favorite pair of jeans.

I then explain that they must put them on, looking at themselves objectively in the mirror.
They should remember to look at themselves objectively in the mirror and in their mind reshaping their body.

It is important to do this when alone, making absolutely sure nobody sees them doing this.

How come?

Since in the beginning it is obvious these clothes do not fit, some people are quick to give unpleasant comments while starting to put these clothes on. They may be good at giving their opinion on the method they use for getting slimmer.

So now, how about you?

Are you ready to prove to your mind you mean business, that you truly want the great pleasure of slimming down in a healthy way?

If the answer is yes, look at yourself in the mirror with the clothes in the size you will wear and in your mind redesign your body as you are assessing what part of your body must change to be able to wear comfortably what you are now uncomfortable wearing or no longer able to enjoy.

- No judgment
- No criticism
- No guilt
- No nothing

Just look at yourself and mentally reshape your body.

As you probably noticed, I keep mentioning "the pleasure of slimming down in a healthy way."

The subconscious mind is lazy and will use the path of least resistance to get to the size you want to be. There are many ways to lose weight. It is important that you *focus* on the pleasure of it as well as keeping your *focus* on slimming down in a healthy way to do so.

Once you start to slim down, you will notice you will do so at a pace that allows your skin to stay smooth, clinging nicely on your body.

Do you want to have the pleasure of slimming down in a healthy way? Of course! Just remain private with what you are doing, only suggesting a person to buy the book should they wonder about what got you in good shape, and let them have their own opinion.

In your mind's eye, it is important to have the pleasure of seeing yourself the way you want to look. It is the only physical exercise you will have to do, to prove to your mind you mean business.

No criticism, only having a good look at yourselves in an objective way. Looking at yourself in the mirror to decide what has to slim down first. In your mind, reshape your body so the jeans can reach the waist (for example).

Once that goal is reached, the next step is followed by being able to button them up. No criticism. In your mind, looking in the mirror, reshape your body.

Once that goal is reached, the next step is being comfortable wearing them.

Humour helps a lot. Make a point of having fun as you mentally reshape your body, and this in the privacy of your own mind.

Please do as I do: Take notes. When a client comes to my office requesting a private session to lose weight, I ask them to do these steps:

Complete the self-assessment about what is constantly on your mind when it comes to your body shape. What are you obsessed about? Do this honestly.

Since writing things down by hand impresses your mind, you will have better results when writing this by hand.

It is important for you to check your progress regularly.

Please remember to write the current date each time you record your findings.

You can get a complementary copy of these questions and all the questions in this book including space to write in a downloadable PDF file at:

http://www.connectwithanny.com

Today's date: _____

(1) What size of shirt are you wearing now?

_____

(2) What size of shirt would you like to wear?

_____

(3) What size of jacket are you wearing now?

_____

(4) What size of jacket would you like to wear?

_____

(5) What size of pants are you wearing now?

_____

(6) What size of pants you would like to wear?

_____

And for ladies:

(7) What size of dress are you wearing now?

_____

(8) What size of dress would you like to wear?

_____

(9) What size of skirt are you wearing now?

_____

(10) What size of skirt would you like to wear?

_____

(11) Write down the clothes you loved so much to wear and you kept, although they no longer fit:

_____

_____

It is important for you to check your progress regularly.

Please remember to write the current date each time you record your findings.

Today's date: _____

(1) What size of shirt are you wearing now?

_____

(2) What size of shirt would you like to wear?

_____

(3) What size of jacket are you wearing now?

_____

(4) What size of jacket would you like to wear?

_____

(5) What size of pants are you wearing now?

_____

 (6) What size of pants you would like to wear?

_____

And for ladies:

(7) What size of dress are you wearing now?

_____

(8) What size of dress would you like to wear?

_____

(9) What size of skirt are you wearing now?

_____

(10) What size of skirt would you like to wear?

_____

(11) Write down the clothes you loved so much to
     wear and you kept, although they no longer
     fit:

_____

_____

It is important for you to check your progress
regularly.

Please remember to write the current date each time
you record your findings.

Today's date: _____

(1) What size of shirt are you wearing now?
_____

(2) What size of shirt would you like to wear?
_____

(3) What size of jacket are you wearing now?

_____

(4) What size of jacket would you like to wear?

_____

(5) What size of pants are you wearing now?

_____

(6) What size of pants you would like to wear?

_____

And for ladies:

(7) What size of dress are you wearing now?

_____

(8) What size of dress would you like to wear?

_____

(9) What size of skirt are you wearing now?

_____

(10) What size of skirt would you like to wear?

_____

(11) Write down the clothes you loved so much to
     wear and you kept, although they no longer
     fit:

_____

_____

It is important for you to check your progress
regularly.

Please remember to write the current date each time
you record your findings.

======================================

THE THIRD MENTAL AGREEMENT

THE MENTAL BLOCKS

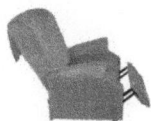

======================================

THE THIRD MENTAL AGREEMENT

Your wants will come upon the conditions you put them on.

Ramtha, the Ram

UNDERSTANDING THE MENTAL BLOCK RESOLVING THE CONFLICT WITHIN

- WHAT IS IT?
- WHO DOES IT?
- WHAT FOR?
- WHAT SIGNALS A MENTAL BLOCK?
- HOW TO REMOVE IT

Do you have a vehicle?

If the front tire on the passenger's side keeps wearing out in an unusual way, what would you do?

Would you keep replacing it with a new tire, or go to the shop and ask the mechanic to check what causes the tire to wear out that way? Right?

You know you must go to the cause of the problem in order to fix it.

The next step is to fix it or repair it. Knowing what the problem is lets you know what you are dealing with. However, unless the problem is solved, it will still be there.

The same goes with everything, including your weight. Your inner work starts once you know what the mental block is all about, followed by resolving that decision in time.

This is a fascinating and conscious journey within. It will reveal it is not what you eat that makes you fat. It is what makes you eat, that decision frozen in time, that makes you fat.

It is true that you will start to slim down by just improving your *focus* and seeing yourself wearing the size of clothes you want to wear.

However, just like having to keep replacing the tire, you will have to keep doing it or the mental block will put you back to square one.

This is just like losing weight by following a diet. Stop the diet and the weight comes back.

What is the block in your head? That decision back in time about your body that keeps running your life, no matter what you do?

By removing the mental block (that outdated decision frozen in time), you will be on full automatic, slimming down and staying slim.

Known to sales managers as the comfort zone, a mental block is a decision made at a time of high emotion.

What do I mean? Let me give you an example.

At one point, a person manages to make a good living and it looks like their income that year will be better than before.
However, once having reached the usual yearly income, something happens (illness, lay-off, company shutting down one of their departments, and more). At the end of the year, the income is the same as before.

Without even being consciously aware of it, this decision can impact your life drastically.

The mental block usually shows up as a symptom such as weight, hiding the cause, the decision made in the past.

To remove the mental block requires teamwork with a therapist, the inner self who made the decision such as weight frozen in time, and the client who comes for sessions.

Who is the boss at this point of time, the part of you from the past who made the decision to experience what you are experiencing now, or you who is reading this now?

How come is it so important to go into the past when we deal with the present?

Having to use willpower signals a major conflict between the parts of you: That younger you whose mind was impressed with the decision you want to update, and you now. This part of you (usually stubborn) sets up a fight, knowing the decision and the perceived benefit will be dismissed.

This is the reason it takes several sessions to have the cooperation of the part of you who made the outdated decision in the past to let go of the perceived benefit and accept your decision in the now.

Weight loss worries

Nurses who come to see me to slim down taught me a very valuable lesson about all this.

For some people, losing weight unconsciously equals being sick. As a result, this creates a powerful mental block. Having observed a terminally ill loved one losing weight creates a fear, sabotaging their efforts to be slim.

Many times, for a nurse, being slim equals death! Now THAT is a mental block!

We are all frozen at different stages of maturity. Through our emotional development, as we live and experience our lives, we imprint ourselves with many subconscious decisions and perceptions.

These decisions create a pattern of response and even form our perceptions of current events and activities.

These decisions made in time are a mental block that creates a perceived comfort zone, feeling safe, regardless of how outdated it is.

What signals a mental block at play?
Having to use willpower signals a major conflict within yourself.

How do we resolve it and who can help us do so?
The first thing is to be aware of how we respond to a situation.

As an instructor, I can see it clearly when giving a course in a school in a continuing education program.

The school bench instantly becomes a catalyst as the students subconsciously find themselves back to a time at school.

This is a mental block at play. It makes me smile as I observe some students starting to re-enact themselves at a much younger age than they are now.

To my observation, the only way to improve any situation is to go from now back to the moment of decision.

Therefore, you must connect and establish rapport with the younger inner person to understand what the situation was that impressed their mind. Once having understood what was going on according to them, simply update the inner younger person and then get their cooperation so the decision can be improved to what is needed in the present.

Having obtained the cooperation of both the inner younger self and the client in the now,
then comes the deal working with two people.

The client in the recliner, and the same person defined as "the inner self," who decided whatever it is the client wants to improve now.

Since the inner self is stuck in their decision, having established a mental block, ready for an argument, staying put, it is important to establish a good rapport with the inner-self so they listen to the views of the person in the now.

Understand that the client finds themselves at two different stages in their life: The then and the now. Discovering when a decision was made to look a certain way, and the "what for" was a valid decision that made sense to the inner-self at that point in time, and is outdated for the person now makes a person realise what is the real issue they are dealing with, allowing them to slim down.

The interesting part is the decision of how to look can have been made at any time:

- In a past life
- Still in the spirit form observing the future mother and her partner having sex or making love
- just before conception
- in the womb
- at birth
- as a child
- a pre-teen
- a teenager
- an adult.

It takes a good therapist to work with mental blocks, to be able to observe what is unfolding, stay, out of the drama, and make sure they think only "I wonder what it is."

That is done by only asking open-ended questions and staying out of what is unfolding. A question that includes an answer is a leading question, making the person respond the way the therapist feels the question should be answered.

This, by the way, is how false memory is created. It can also be created when you are in shock, frightened, intimidated, or anaesthetised.

Please pay attention to the way people are interviewed on the radio or TV and notice how the hosts ask the questions. Many lead the guests to answer the way they think the answer should be. You will then clearly understand the difference between a leading question and an open-ended question.

Should you find yourself in a situation when there is no therapist to help you with this, I offer this service literally at a distance. I will connect with you wherever you are on this planet. This is called "virtual hypnotherapy sessions." Information about this service can be found by visiting:
http:// www.success-and-more.com/services.html

Here are some examples to help you understand the creation of a mental block, and the resulting inner fight, of having to use willpower to accomplish what you desire.

Smoking

During one of my weeklong hypnotherapy trainings, the class asked me to do a demonstration regarding stop smoking.

A student volunteered who wanted to quit smoking.

Once in an hypnotic trance and in a superconscious state, the session quickly led the student to the decision to first smoke at the age of fourteen. I immediately had a furious teenager to deal with. Yelling and screaming in teenage rebellion, the student started to rant about how her mother had kicked her beloved father out of the house—and this, without asking her opinion. How dare she!

She decided to smoke to punish her mother in a way that would make her mother very angry.

She locked herself in the bathroom, opened the bathroom window, and started to smoke heavily, one cigarette after another, making sure the smoke could be seen coming out of the window—not to mention the odour that filled the bathroom and a good part of the house once she opened the bathroom door.

She had smoked ever since, deep down at subconscious level still enjoying her mother's objections – Mission successfully carried out!

I then asked the student in the present who wanted to quit smoking to review and explain the situation to the fourteen-year-old inner self, making her understand from her current position the point of view that made her mother decide to kick the father out of the house.

Having the approved co-operation of the inner fourteen-year-old, I then gave her the choice:

When did she want to quit smoking?
- Right now? (it was Monday)
- By Friday night?
- By Sunday night?

The inner fourteen-year-old returned yelling: "This is ridiculous! I want to quit right now!"

When I asked the student in the present when she wanted to quit smoking, she said,

"This coming Friday night."

Who do you think is the boss, the fourteen-year-old who made the decision to smoke in the first place and then changed her mind and decided it is time to quit right now, or the student in present time who wanted to quit smoking the coming Friday night?

During the balance of the weeklong course, coming to class, the student complained every day that she wanted to smoke and was unable to do so. The fourteen-year-old was in charge!

Let me give you a second example:

Business income

Many years ago, I realised my business income was the same for three years in a row, no matter what I was doing.

This was a mental block about my business income, a comfort zone.

Walking my talk and knowing I train the best, I decided to have a hypnotherapy session with one of the excellent hypnotherapists trained by me.

Once in a hypnotic trance, I quickly found myself back in Congo at twenty-five years of age, saying goodbye to Papa as my husband and I were leaving for Canada.

Papa had an excellent business. One of his successful practices was to reinvest into his business as it grew, and it grew into one of the best in his trade.

As we looked at each other, knowing deep down that we would not see each other again, in my hypnotic trance I discovered that I thought:

"What is the point of working so hard when someone will take it away from you?"

Without realising it, this observation created a mental block. I experienced what was happening to my father. He built a successful business only to lose it all due to political upheaval.

The session then went quickly, my hypnotherapist keeping me on track, listening to me as I was explaining to my much younger self that we live now in Canada, a country stable and very different from the Congo. There, the indigenous were taking and looting everything since their independence.

A few weeks later, I went to the bank to pay:

- My personal income tax
- My husband's income tax
- Canada corporation tax
- Provincial corporation tax
- Payroll deductions
- Goods and Services Tax)

As the teller at the bank was stamping the slips and the corresponding cheques, she said,

"The government: They take all our money away!"

I spontaneously replied:
"That is fine. There is a lot of money left!"

I realised the mental block was dissolved and knew my business would flourish as I meant it to be.

Weight - "That's not my father!"

A lady came to lose weight, wondering how come all her siblings were slender just like her father and she looked and was plump like her mother.

Superconscious and in a hypnotic trance, she found herself just before conception observing her mother and her father making love.

My client kept repeating that she had never felt such a deep and profound love in her life.

Totally wrapped into that passionate profound deep love, all of a sudden, I noticed her eyes wide open beneath her closed eyelids as she recognised the man and exclaimed,
"That is not my father!"

At that instant and seconds before conception, completely overwhelmed and engulfed in that incredible love between the man and her mother, she decided to look like her mother to protect her mother and her biological father's identity.

After the session, the identity of her biological father was confirmed by family members.

My client knew the man and now understood the pleasant and loving fatherly relationship she had with him. Respecting her mother's secret, my client only allowed herself to slim down after the death of her mother.

Weight - "Just like Grandma."

I remember this session clearly. It was a good twenty-five years ago.

Having done everything to no avail, a client came to see me for a hypnotherapy session, wanting to lose weight.

In a hypnotic trance, she found herself at a young age. There was no love at home, her parents being heavy drinkers. On school days, she would get up early, get dressed, take what she needed for school, and run at her beloved grandmother's place, who lived only two doors away.

She would open the unlocked door, walk in the living room, and was going to bed on the couch in the living room, made ready for her with pillow and blanket.

When it was time to get up to go to school, her grandmother would gently wake her up, having breakfast ready for her.

As my client was lovingly remembering that time, I asked her what was on her mind.

The little inner-self answered:
"I want to be just like Grandma."

I asked my client to open here eyes and stay in a deep trance, gave her paper and pencil, and asked her to draw her grandmother with herself next to her.

The grandmother was very much overweight and so was the little inner-self.

Gently removing paper and pencil, I suggested to my client to close her eyes and return to a very special state of relaxation.

When asked what was it about Grandma that she wanted to be just like her, the little inner-self replied, "She is so nice and kind, I want to be just like her."

Updating the little inner-self as well as my client back into an hypnotic trance, I then explained that she was indeed as nice as loving as Grandma, and that she could be so and be slimmer than her. Yes, she could because she wanted to be as nice and kind as her, and she was.

It took some more explanation until both the inner-self and my client in the recliner were in accord.

It took only that session for my client to slim down in a healthy way.

We are truly one of a kind and I could write a thick book explaining the mental block of each client who came to lose weight, wanting to slim down in a healthy way.

However, I decided not to write such a book because each of us has enough "what for" mental blocks as is!

Like it or not, we must go back to the point of decision, to the formation of the mental block to address any situation.

Money, relationships, behavior, lifestyle, health, illness, everything, including our looks and weight.

Whatever it was that made sense then, many times will make no sense now.

Just like a tire that wears out in an unusual way, we must go to the shop to find what causes the problem and have it fixed to be able to improve any situation.

How come? A decision made with emotion is something that impressed our mind, becomes familiar and becomes our comfort zone, our autopilot.

The perceived one-time benefit (Let us be honest, it works, or we would not keep on doing it again and again) at the time of decision keeps it alive, creating a battle within when using willpower to address a new situation in an outdated response. Many times, a good hypnotherapist can help their client make this journey from effect back to cause, bringing enlightenment, resulting in understanding themselves, and delivering much needed peace of mind.

How do you know you have the pleasure of slimming down in a healthy way?

Simply check how your current clothes are fitting and how the ones you used to wear when slimmer are fitting now... and start shopping for new clothes!

Sometimes I tell my clients, "Baggy pants feel great, making you aware you are getting slimmer."

You will notice I keep insisting on the pleasure of slimming down in a healthy way. There are many reasons to slim down. Please make sure you want the pleasure to do so in a healthy way.

The number of hypnotherapy sessions you will require to slim down in a healthy way depends of the level of acceptance of the inner- self.
The more stubborn it is, the more sessions will be required. The client knows when it is time to come back for more sessions to improve anything, slimming down included.

The body knows at what steady pace to slim down to allow your skin the time to tighten up and hug your body. Therefore, some clients will slim down much slower than others do, allowing their skin to stay tight around their body, depending how much they want to slim down.

==================================

THE FOURTH MENTAL AGREEMENT

WALKING YOUR TALK

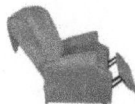

==================================

THE FOURTH MENTAL AGREEMENT

Insanity:
Doing the same thing over and over again
and expecting different results.

Albert Einstein.

WALKING YOUR TALK

"If you always do what you've always done, you always get what you've always gotten." That was the advice of Jessie Potter, the featured speaker at Friday's opening of the seventh annual Woman to Woman conference.

This chapter is set up for journaling and self-assessment. The purpose is for you to stay on the right path, have the pleasure of slimming down in pleasant and healthy way, and stay slim.

Date: _____

(1) What is on your mind as you look at yourself in the mirror?

_____

(2) What do you keep *focusing* on when buying groceries?

_____

(3) Do you regularly put on the size of clothes you want to wear?

_____

(4) When doing so, do you re-shape your body so what you want to wear fits well?

_____

How about looking back at the questions you answered in:

☐ The first mental agreement
The *focus.*

☐ The second mental agreement
Defining the boundaries.

And now

☐ The fourth mental agreement
Walking your talk.

Date:

_____

(1) What is on your mind as you look at yourself in the mirror?

_____

(2) What do you keep *focusing* on when buying groceries?

_____

(3) Do you regularly put on the size of clothes you want to wear?

_____

(4) When doing so, do you re-shape your body so what you want to wear fits well?

_____

How about looking back at the questions you answered in:

☐ The first mental agreement
   The *focus*.

☐ The second mental agreement
   Defining the boundaries.

And now

☐ The fourth mental agreement
   Walking your talk.

Date: _____

(1) What is on your mind as you look at yourself in the mirror?

_____

(2) What do you keep *focusing* on when buying groceries?

_____

(3) Do you regularly put on the size of clothes you want to wear?

_____

(4) When doing so, do you re-shape your body so what you want to wear fits well?

_____

How about looking back at the questions you answered in:

☐ The first mental agreement
The *focus*.

☐ The second mental agreement
Defining the boundaries.

And now

☐ The fourth mental agreement
Walking your talk.

It is important for you to check your progress regularly

Please remember to write the current date each time you record your findings.

You can get a complementary copy of these questions and all the questions in this book including space to write in a downloadable PDF file at:

http://www.connectwithanny.com

YOUR BRAIN NEEDS ATTENTION TOO

Being slim does not mean being healthy.

The title of this book is:
The Four Mental Agreements to Losing Weight.

Everything is mental, using your mind.

By now, you must have noticed that I keep talking about the mind, that non-physical part of us.

Have you ever thought how come we can see something in our mind and it manifests?

Dr. Wilder Penfield (1891-1976) was one of the greatest neuroscientists who ever lived.

A Canadian, Dr. Penfield, after years of research, discovered and confirmed the mind is not physical and has a different function than the brain, that physical part of us.

We are more than flesh and bones.
The mind, our thoughts, are non-physical and the brain is physical.

Therefore, the mind needs a fully functional brain to successfully "download" information or a command.

The command is a perception you can describe; a picture the mind sends to the brain.

Although physical, the function of the brain is truly magical.

This is the reason I am asking you to look at yourself in the mirror, reshaping your body to your liking and to allow yourself to fit comfortably in the clothes you want to wear.

Can you read French? If so, may I strongly suggest the book, *L'erreur de Broca, Exploration d'un cerveau éveillé*, by Professor Hugues Duffau, neurosurgeon at the CHU of Montpellier, France.

In his book, Professor Duffau praises Dr. Wilder Penfield (1891-1976) for his findings about the workings of the brain.
It is a fascinating read. I hope this book will soon be translated in English for you all to read.

Upon the diagnosis that her daughter had a brain tumor, one of my sisters did some research to know how come her daughter had a malignant brain tumor after having lost a breast to cancer a few years before.

My sister found the answer, reading an old book printed in 1929.

The information in that book is a gem and if you can read French, I recommend you get a copy.

In *Le Chemin Du Bonheur, La Rééducation De Soi-même* (loosely translated as The Way to Happiness, The Re-education of Self), by Dr. Victor Pauchet, the author explained:

Being constipated or when holding a bowel movement "until later," all the toxins the body wants to expel stay in the body, poisoning it.

In his book, Dr. Victor Pauchet explained by his observation that not expelling the toxins is the major cause of cancer and brain tumours, and suspected it is also the major cause of many other ailments.

For example, bladder infections affect the brain, resulting in loss of cognition.

It is also important to make sure that whatever you ingest, the liver can process it and stay intact in the process.

Dr. Pauchet also explains that the digestion process starts with salivation as we eat, followed by chewing the food as we savour it.

By reading Dr. Pauchet's book, I also wonder how fast food influences how many people eat, as well as their resulting health and looks.

Here in Canada, when in a restaurant, the waiter or waitress removes immediately the plate of the person who has finished their meal while other guests are slow and still eating.

As I see it, this is a subtle suggestion to the other guests that they want them to speed up and leave the restaurant to have a table for other patrons.

I am not a medical doctor and there is no doubt that illnesses may be caused by other sources. However, in my view, this basic health information is part of an effective preventive maintenance program.

To your health!,

Anny.

THE RECIPE, DIET, AND EXERCISE PAGE

"New and stirring things are belittled because if they are not belittled the humiliating question arises 'Why then are you not taking part in them?"

- H.G. Wells

At the last count, having shared a draft of the book with over thirty people, asking for their comments, it was explained that sometimes there is resistance to the words "slimming down."

For example, for an athletic person, slimming down means losing body fat and getting weak. In this instance, "fit, strong, and healthy" would be a more correct term.

Therefore, please adjust the term "slimming down" to an affirmation that you will subconsciously accept.

It will work as long as you have the correct *focus* in mind: Looking the way you want to look.

Going to the gym to exercise to look good and attract your soulmate (or swolemate, to use the gym jargon) is great.

Swole is slang for "swollen." It's just a term to describe that pumped up feeling or appearance you get from working out.

Swolemate is another popular hashtag that refers to a workout partner or inspirational person.

I observed that once they are swolemates, they train together to achieve a common goal.

That is right:

You and your **SWOLEMATE** *grow together, both literally and figuratively.*

Once the goal has been reached, the *focus* changes and it is all fun and games until the jeans do not fit anymore.

In conclusion, regardless of what you are *focusing* on, the mental blocks frozen in time, will have the day and run the show.

When the mental blocks about your weight and looks have been resolved, you will run the show!

It is not what you eat that makes you fat, it is what makes you eat that makes you fat.

This book is a self-help book. I have included many important examples that may seem unrelated to you, to help you understand what a *focus* is as well as the creation and role of a mental block.

Your *focus* and the mental blocks are the only two issues you have to resolve to allow yourself to slim down in a healthy way, and stay slim.

Remember: Keep doing what you do and you keep having what you have.

If you think there should be recipes, diet plans, and exercise regimens here, you have misunderstood the *focus* of this book.

To have the complete benefit, please adjust your *focus* and re-read the book from cover to cover.

"The person who says something is impossible should not interrupt the person who is doing it."

- Chinese Proverb

Thoughts are things. They materialise.

Wishing you the pleasure to succeed in all your endeavors.

Sincerely,

Anny

AFTERWORD

As you are reviewing the questions in Chapter 4, I hope you realise the information is about more than just slimming down in a healthy way.

As you are taking note of what is explained in this book, I am giving you more than a way to slim down in a pleasant, easy, and healthy way. The same four steps apply for your life experiences.

1 Your focus.
2 Seeing it in your mind.
3 Deep down allowing you
to be and do so.

and then,

4 Walking your talk.

What is true for you to design your body is also true for defining what you want your life to be.

The focus, seeing the results in your mind's eye are the most important things you do.

First, the focus. Just like for slimming down, are you focusing on how to get "it" instead of having the pleasure of having what you want?

Focusing on the "how to" is an excellent way to accomplish nothing since the focus is the "how to" instead of the result.

Have you used willpower to get what you want? The next step is to get qualified help to remove the mental block, that decision made back in time to allow yourself the pleasure to get what you want at present time.

Let me give you some example:

Walking back home

How did my father in-law walk back home from a German concentration camp?

During World War II, my father in-law was turned in as a saboteur and a spy working for the underground army.

I am using the phrase "turned in" since it is a local man who advised the Germans about it, the Germans having no clue.

He was first held in a special facility in Belgium, where he was beaten and tortured in an attempt to get him to give them the names of the other members of the underground army —and this to no avail.

Being arrested as a spy, how come he was sent to working concentration camps in Germany and not executed, and how did he survive?

He was in working concentration camps in Sangerhauzen, Buchenwald, Dora, Harzengen, and Beedorf.

At one point while in a concentration camp, a German guard observed him only eating charcoal, as my father in-law knew it cures severe diarrhea.

A German guard then gave him medication telling him, "Here, we know you want to live."

After the liberation, exhausted, weak, and having lost a tremendous amount of weight from all the time in concentration camps at liberation, my father in-law walked out of the camp he was in.

The prisoners were marching on the road, doing what they called "La Marche à la Mort." Loosely translated, it meant march or die.

They all ended up free, the German guards having run for their lives as the Allies were flying very close to the ground, cockpit open, waving at the prisoners, ready to shoot down anyone not wearing the prisoner's uniform.

It was explained to me that the planes were flying so low over the road that the few cars on the road would suddenly leave the road in fear the planes would land on the road, hit and crush them.

As they were marching, my father-in-law's group came across an abandoned German truck and quickly found out what mechanical part was missing.

Born and raised in Belgium close to the German border, my father-in-law spoke German fluently.

The sabotaged truck was parked in front of a house. He went to the house and asked for the part.

The man did not want to give it to him, upon which my father-in-law produced a hand gun he was carrying (Yes, some highly trusted prisoners managed to have hand guns while in concentration camp—unknown to the Germans, of course).

The German's wife then said, 'Give it to him.'

The truck was repaired and back on the road, loaded to extra full capacity with liberated prisoners.

They parted once in Belgium and my father in- law walked to one of his wife's brother's home, who immediately called my husband's mother to let her know he was back, and drove him to a clinic run by one of my father in-law's own brother-in-law, a medical doctor.

After several weeks in his brother-in-law's clinic to get some strength and some of his health back, my father in-law was driven back home.

He was helped getting out of the car and walked, entering his house.

He walked back home.

How come?

Once back home, he explained that while in concentration camps, all what he was focusing on was walking back home, and in his mind's eye, seeing himself doing so.

A second example from a colleague:

On a lake, caught in a storm

Finding himself in a sudden threatening storm while canoeing on a lake here in Canada, in his mind's eye he threw a rope attached to his canoe to the place he had planned to reach.

Then in his mind, he made sure it was attached to a firmly anchored winch.

Paddling furiously, battling huge waves, his focus remaining only on the place he had planned to reach. He made it, exhausted, safe and sound, and soaking wet.

Just like my father in-law focusing on walking back home and my colleague focusing on the place he had planned to reach, what is your focus about your weight?

ONLINE STORE, CONTACT, AND MORE

You may contact Anny by visiting any of her websites and scroll down the home page to the contact information.

http://www.annyslegten.com
> Her private website
> Online store

http://www.success-and-more.com
> To find the description of the services offered, and more.

http://www.htialberta.com
> The Hypnotism Training Institute of Alberta website

http://www.reiki-canada.com
> About the Reiki Training Centre of Canada

http://www.slegtenianhypnosis.com
> Although open to anyone interested in this fascinating hypnosis modality, this website information is for the Hypnotism Training Institute of Alberta graduates.

HYPNOTHERAPY, A HEALING MODALITY

There are many healing resources. The choice will be governed by how fast one wants to advance in life.

As a hypnotherapist, I understand that the reason a person seeks help is usually a symptom of something different, many times seemingly out of context and only making sense to the client.

Hypnosis can be done over the telephone. However, for hypnotherapy, using hypnosis to facilitate therapy, personal contact is necessary. There are many nonverbal communications like a tremor in the voice, facial expressions, shifting as we talk, and even physical odour that has nothing to do with hygiene that allow the hypnotherapist to understand and effectively help the client.

From the results clients are reporting, a virtual hypnotherapy session is by far the most potent. During a virtual (sometimes called surrogate) session, we are in fact reading the client in a way that can be experienced only in that modality.

In my experience, the purpose of the session is an investigation or healing session for everyone concerned. Reading a client with my five senses, I then switch and become the hypnotherapist.

When doing the deep trance hypnotherapy, reading in front of the person who requested the healing, much energy is required to constantly block the client's thoughts, to get a pure answer. The best and most effective results are by far doing the session while the person is absent, not knowing the day and time their session will be performed. Whether a one-on-one hypnotherapy session or a hypnotherapy session at a distance by surrogate, the number of sessions depends on the client.

In my experience, any work involving what one would call a mental illness may require up to four surrogate hypnotherapy sessions, occasionally more, to clear the emotional cause leading to the physical symptoms. During a surrogate hypnotherapy reading session, all information comes from a nonphysical source.

I am not a physician, and I do not claim to heal any medical condition. Over the years, I learned that the way a person was told of their physical condition can be the catalyst of the outcome. I only do whatever is possible for my clients to shift into the results they are seeking.

Yes, as potent as a one on one hypnotherapy session or surrogate hypnotherapy reading session is, only the client can make the necessary shift. No one, not even me, can do it for them.

Complete information on this subject can be found by visiting **http://www.success-and-more.com/services.html**

Having never experienced being in a hypnotic trance that they are aware of, some people have an interesting idea of what being hypnotised is.

As explained before, no matter what, the person in a hypnotic trance is always in total control. Yes, a person can lie through their teeth if they choose to do so.

Not feeling safe by having a one on one hypnotherapy session or a virtual hypnotherapy session, a person asked if meditation would work too.

There is a difference between hypnosis and meditation, which is noticed by brainwaves during hypnosis and meditation by HZ, or cycles/second.

Hypnosis shows a much slower cycle than meditation.

Voltage between head and other parts of the body become more negative during physical activity, decline in sleep, and reverse to positive under general anaesthesia.

It is a change in voltage.

Information from:
The Body Electric
By Roberts O. Becker, MD and Gary Selden

To my understanding, meditation connects with the brain and hypnosis allows us to connect with the mind.

Do you wonder how come I have a picture of my recliner printed on some pages?

After all, it is only a recliner, or so you may think!

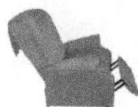

At the end of a highly emotional and delightful hypnotherapy session involving his relationship with his father, a man in his mid-twenties got up and, pointing to my recliner said, "This is a magic chair!"

Since then, the picture of my recliner has been my trademark.

I recently had to put it in retirement, worn out after thirty-one years of constant use. I had to hold the back of the recliner for fear of the chair flipping back to the floor when put in the recliner position.

It is with relief that I observe the new recliner has taken over the magic side of the hypnotherapy sessions.

DESCRIPTIONS OR GLOSSARY

Cognition:

Losing awareness and judgment.
May cause a person to lose their balance.

Focus:

The concentration of attention on a specific outcome.

Hypnology:

The study of hypnosis in all its forms and applications.

Hypnosis, Hypnotherapy:

Hypnosis is a technique connecting with the brain, which is the reason it has to be repeated over and over again.

To my understanding, hypnotherapy is a technique to connect with the mind, bypassing the brain. Hypnotherapy requires more training. It uses hypnosis, the tool, to do therapy.

For example, hypnosis is used during childbirth to relax and experience a comfortable and natural birthing experience. By bypassing the brain and connecting with the mind, the client becomes super conscious, finding themselves both in the past and in the now, and in a conscious hypnotic trance, they go to the cause of the symptom they are dealing with, being emotional or physical.

Hypnotism Training Institute of Alberta

The hypnosis school run by Anny Slegten. In Canada, a school denotes a teaching business, not a building where you go to school.

Mental blocks

Having to use willpower to achieve anything signals a fixed idea. It is a decision or observation made earlier in time about the subject matter.

At the time, it was the best decision we could have made. Lodged at subconscious level, it will fight for its survival, no matter outdated at present time.

It is a defense mechanism to keep things "Status quo", maintaining the subject matter in its existing state.

Penfield, Wilder

Wilder Penfield (1891–1976) was the founder of the Montreal Neurological Institute, and one of the greatest neuroscientists who ever lived. In his many research experiments, Penfield reported that there is no place in the cerebral cortex where electrical stimulation will cause a patient to believe, decide, or have will. These are not functions of brain, but of the "I," or soul.

The brain is physical and is connected to the physical body. The mind is nonphysical and is connected to the soul.

ABOUT THE AUTHOR

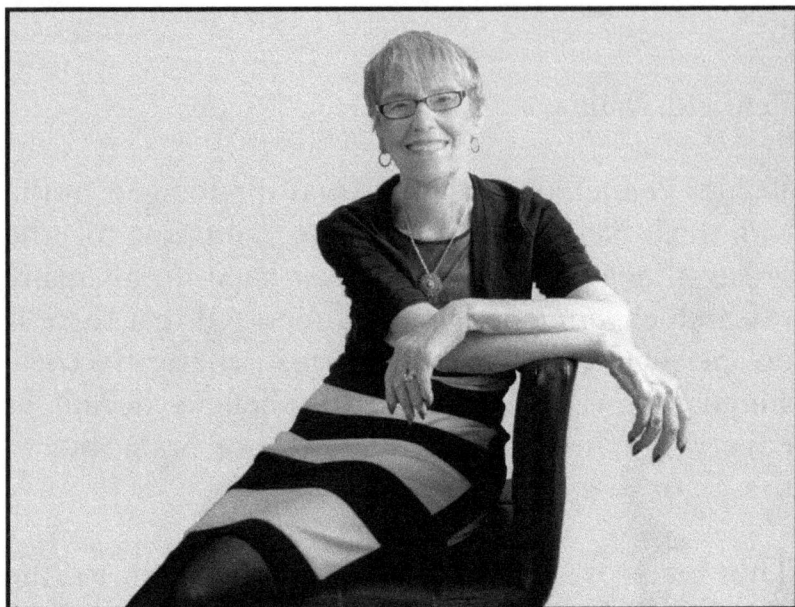

Having experienced life in three continents, observing hundreds of different cultures and ways of thinking, Anny Slegten has developed a universal way of perceiving life, specialising on removing mental blocks.

Anny is continually searching to understand the Universal Energy that bonds everything together.

A hypnotist, hypnotherapist, hypnologist, Hypno-Baby-Birthing facilitator, Reiki master/teacher, master remote viewer, and author, Anny Slegten is a world renowned clinical hypnotherapist and hypnologist in full time practice since 1984.

Director of The Hypnotism Training Institute of Alberta, Anny developed and structured the training and curriculum to the highest standards and offers training to students that come from around the globe.

Wondering how Anny Slegten got into this?

You may find the information by visiting her personal website at:

http://www.annyslegten.com

Other books by Anny Slegten

Other books published by Anny Slegten can be found at:

https://www.annyslegten.com/books

as well as ordering on Amazon when deciding to buy a book.

www.ingramcontent.com/pod-product-compliance
Lightning Source LLC
Chambersburg PA
CBHW030021290326
41934CB00005B/428